CONQUERING INTERMITTENT FASTING

HOW TO SAY "NO" TO YOURSELF

By **M.L. PILGRIM**

TO MY WIFE AND MY SON, THIS BOOK
IS FOR YOU.

Copyright

Disclaimer

All intellect contained in this book is given for enlightening and instructive purposes as it were. The creator isn't in any capacity responsible for any outcomes or results that radiate from utilising this material. Worthwhile endeavours have been made to give data that is both precise and viable. However, the creator isn't oriented for the exactness or use/misuse of this data.

Table of Contents

Introduction

Without a doubt, intermittent fasting does not only help you lose weight, but it also clears your mind and gives you more energy. But where do you start?

With the Basics

This book teaches you about intermittent fasting with quick and easy plans to understand. Are you wondering how to set up your fasts? You will find out how to systematically plan your eating habits. Not sure how to get the most out of this practice? You will see a clear set of guidelines, including various fasting plans, so you can choose the one that best suits your schedule and needs. Not sure how to work out a diet that works best with intermittent fasting? This book offers detailed advice on what to eat and drink. In addition, there are over fifty delicious recipes that will complement your fasting in a healthy way.

You will learn the pros and cons of fasting. The way you apply this information is up to you. You may want to establish a regular fasting program, or you may want to spontaneously fast when the time is right. Maybe you want to lose weight while dealing with health problems?

Whatever the reason for intermittent fasting, this book is here to help you safely adopt this new lifestyle and apply it to your life, simply and effectively.

CHAPTER ONE-Getting Started with Intermittent Fasting

As the name suggests, intermittent fasting is a lifestyle that periodically goes without food. This does not mean that you are starving, far from it. Instead, combine fasting with a healthy diet, keeping in mind what you eat and drink to promote better health and mental clarity. If properly addressed, intermittent fasting can help you fight diabetes and other conditions related to hyperglycemia, as well as insomnia and heart disease. If you are interested in intermittent fasting, the following guidelines can help you get started.

What is Intermittent Fasting?

Even though you seem to have heard of it much more recently, intermittent fasting is not a new concept. Indeed, fasting has been an important part of history and religion for centuries. Many people begin to understand the health benefits of fasting, whether it's more energy, weight loss, or greater mental clarity. Intermittent fasting is not a specific diet. This is a general term that describes a way of eating where you alternate between eating and fasting (voluntarily depriving yourself of food for a certain period of time). To fully understand intermittent fasting, it is useful to know the difference between a fed state and a fasting state: the two phases of the digestive system.

The Fed State

A NUTRITIONAL or absorbent state occurs immediately after a meal or snack when your body digests food and absorbs its nutrients. Digestion continues until the decomposed components of the food are transported through the blood, where they go to the liver, fatty tissues, and muscles.

Decomposed food that first enters the blood increases blood sugar, which then stimulates beta cells (the specialized cells in the pancreas that produce, store, and release insulin) to release insulin into the blood. The released insulin binds to glucose in the blood and directs it to the cells, where it is used as an energy source, or to the liver and muscles, where it is converted into glycogen and stored for use.

The Fasted State

Once the nourished state is over, your body goes into a state of fasting or post-absorption. When you fast, about four hours after eating, your body needs stored glycogen for energy. Blood glucose levels decrease when cells start using sugar, and, in response to this decrease in glucose, insulin levels also decrease. Since your body wants to maintain a blood sugar level of between 70 and 99 milligrams per deciliter, this drop in blood glucose causes the hormone alpha cells in the pancreas to discharge a hormone called glucagon. Glucagon goes to the liver, where it separates glycogen into glucose. When glucose is framed, it is discharged from the liver and goes to the cerebrum and tissues.

For what reason do People Fast?

With regard to the historical backdrop of human advancement, simple and normal access to food is really a moderately new idea. Prior to the mechanical transformation, individuals needed to depend exclusively on earth for food. They just couldn't go to the closest grocery store each time they expected to fill their stomachs. Old developments chased and accumulated, however much as could be expected (and a few human advancements around the globe despite everything chase and assemble today). In any case, food hasn't generally been an assurance. Sometimes hunters and gatherers would return with an expedition of fresh fruit and fresh berries; on other days, especially in periods of scarcity, such as the winter months, they returned empty-handed. Although they didn't do it intentionally, they were essentially fasting these days, which entirely is determined by the time of year and the skill of hunters and gatherers, and these fasts can last for days, weeks, or even months.

Fasting in Ancient Times

Some ancient civilizations understood the benefits of fasting long before today. Many greeks believe that intermittent fasting improves cognitive skills and concentration. And according to Benjamin Franklin, one of the founding fathers of the United States and the alleged inventor of the lightning rod and bifocal glasses, the best of all drugs is rest and fasting.

Spiritual Fasting

Fasting has additionally been and keeps on being a significant piece of different strict and profound practices the world over. At the point when utilized for strict purposes, fasting is regularly depicted as a detoxification or cleaning process, yet the essential idea is consistently the equivalent: forgoing eating for a specific timeframe.

In contrast to clinical fasting, which is utilized as a treatment for illness, otherworldly fasting is viewed as a significant impetus for the prosperity of the entire body, and a wide assortment of religions shares the conviction that fasting has the ability to mend.

In Christianity, fasting is a means of purifying the soul so that the body is pure, and a connection to God can be established. One of the most popular times when Christians fast in Lent, the forty-day period between Ash Wednesday and Easter. In the past, those who observed Lent gave up eating or drinking; even today, Christians refrained from eating or drinking, but often chose to do without something specific. This practice is an acknowledgment of the forty days that Jesus Christ spent in the desert, forced to fast.

Perhaps the best known religious fast, Ramadan is an important part of the Muslim religion and the ninth month of the Islamic calendar. During Ramadan, Muslims not only refrain from eating and drinking from sunset to sunrise but also avoid smoking, sex, and any other activity that could be considered a sin. The fasting period and the slight dehydration that occur due to lack of fluids are believed to purify the soul of harmful impurities so that the heart can be redirected to spirituality and removed from earthly desires. Ramadan is considered to be one of the five pillars of Islam.

Medical Fasting

Hippocrates, nicknamed the father of medicine, introduced fasting as a medical therapy for some of his sick patients as early as the 5th century BC. C. One of his famous quotes says that eating when sick makes the disease worse. According to him, fasting helps the body to focus on healing and that forcing food into a medical condition could be harmful to a person's health because instead of giving energy for healing, his body would use all the energy available to digest. On the other hand, if sick patients refrained from eating, the digestive processes would stop, and the body would prioritize natural healing.

Fasting as a Therapy

Some medical fasts allowed only calorie-free tea and water for a month, while others allowed patients to consume between 200 and 500 calories per day. These calories generally come from bread, broths, juices, and milk. Until the 20th century, fasting began to appear in scientific journals as an effective medical therapy for obesity and other diseases; Even then, the benefits have only recently started to make themselves felt.

Eustress: Short-Term Stress

Good stress, also called eustress, is mild stress that most people experience regularly. Rather than being harmful to the body, the eustress inspires him and pushes him to achieve a desired goal or result, and is generally associated with some type of happiness or emotion when that goal is achieved. Examples of eustress include training for a sporting event, working towards a deadline, or training for an upcoming show. Research shows that eustress can actually improve brain function. The distinctive feature of eustress is that it is short-lived. When the goal is achieved, or the project is completed, the eustress disappears, and its cortisol levels decrease and normalize, giving the body time to recover.

Distress: Bad Stress

Bad stress, or what is called heartache, is chronic and unstoppable stress that damages your productivity or interferes with your daily life. Rather than striving to achieve your goals, anguish makes it more difficult to achieve them. Panic maintains high levels of cortisol and adrenaline, which can lead to a weakening of the adrenal glands and problems with normal hormonal signaling. Chronic health problems associated with anxiety include depression, heart disease, weight gain, and increased vulnerability to diseases such as colds and flu. Examples of suffering include toxic romantic relationships, constant stress at work, and trauma or death in the family.

However, since everyone reacts to certain things differently and has a different perspective on life, the line between good and bad stress can be confusing. The best way to determine if a situation is distressing or distressing is to ask yourself a few questions: do you feel challenged but motivated? If so, it's probably good stress. Do you feel overwhelmed, withdrawn, and tired? If so, it's probably serious stress.

Should You Fast?

Fasting is suitable for most healthy people, but for some, it is better not to fast or talk to your doctor before starting a fast. You should not fast if:

- You are pregnant or breastfeeding
- You are severely underweight or malnourished
- You are under eighteen
- You should speak to your doctor before fasting if you have health problems:
- You are taking medication
- You have a history of eating disorders.
- Have cortisol dysregulation or are under significant stress
- You have diabetes (type 1 or type 2)
- You have GERD (Gastroesophageal reflux disease)
- You have gout

Tune in to Your Body!

Listen cautiously to your body to decide whether fasting is directly for you. On the off chance that you feel shy of vitality or discombobulated while on your feet, you may need to modify your fasting period or counsel your primary care physician to ensure your body can direct glucose effectively. Remember that it can, at times, require some investment for your body to adjust to your new way of life. There is typically a three to multi-week progress period during which the body and mind adjust to fasting. During this time, you may encounter hunger, peevishness, shortcoming, and even loss of moxie.

This is a normal reaction, but if the symptoms are severe, consults your doctor during these first steps. If you feel good after the adaptation period, this is a good sign that your body appreciates what it is doing. If, after this period, you feel dizzy, dizzy, or run out of energy, you should stop fasting and talk to your doctor.

Fasting and Diabetes

Diabetic people can find fasting hard because it is more difficult for the body to regulate insulin and blood sugar levels than people without diabetes. However, research shows that intermittent fasting can be helpful in helping to restore blood sugar to a normal level. Hypoglycemia, or hypoglycemia, is the main concern for fasting and diabetes.

If that you have diabetes, ensure you have the specialist's endorsement and management before beginning any sort of quick. If your doctor endorses irregular fasting, acclimate yourself with the side effects of hypoglycemia and plan to treat your glucose level on the off chance that it is excessively low. In the event that the glucose level surpasses 300 milligrams for every deciliter or falls beneath 70 milligrams for each deciliter, quit fasting promptly, and apply the fitting treatment.

Hypoglycemia is more likely in people with type 1 diabetes than in people with type 2 diabetes. Signs of hypoglycemia include:

- Anxiety
- Fatigue
- Hunger/Starvation
- Increased Sweating

- Irregular heartbeat
- Irritability
- Pale skin
- Severe hypoglycemia can cause:
- Abnormal behavior or mental confusion.
- Poor eyesight
- Confusion
- Loss of consciousness

Take Control of Chronic Diseases

The stress that fasting exerts on the body can be classified as Eustress for most people. It is light in weight and generates health benefits that can push you to continue reaching your end goals. However, if you already have chronic discomfort, you will want to check the situation before incorporating intermittent fasting into your daily life. In chronic stress, your body continuously pumps cortisol. When cortisol levels remain elevated for a long time, this can lead to:

- Anxiety
- Depression
- Sleeping difficulty
- Digestive problems
- Headache
- Heart disease
- Memory and concentration problems.
- Weight gain

Over time, chronic stress also negatively affects the function of the adrenal glands and makes it difficult to regulate hormones correctly.

If you are already under severe chronic stress, it is extremely important to have a good understanding of cortisol levels and the proper function of the adrenal glands before starting to fast. You can lower cortisol by meditating, avoiding coffee, getting enough sleep, eating a healthy, clean diet for some time before incorporating fasting, and avoiding excessive exercise. Low impact meditation exercises like yoga can be helpful.

Prepare to Fast

With the exception of spontaneous fasting (which we will discuss later), most intermittent fasting requires preparation. What type of intermittent fasting are you going to do? On what days and hours will you fast? What is your official start date? It is useful to write a program and keep it handy, so you can always see it. You can even set your phone's timers to ring when it's time to start fasting and when it's time to start eating again. But you don't even need to start an established quick program right away; you can gradually get used to taking advantage of it.

Do Yoga

In a study by the Yoga Research Society and Sidney Kimmel Medical College at Thomas Jefferson University, researchers found that cortisol levels dropped significantly after a fifty-minute yoga class that included popular poses such as tree pose, Pose of the snowplow and laying of the locust. This relaxation reaction puts an end to the cascade of stress, and therefore, the stress hormones are naturally reduced. High levels of cortisol are also common in depressed people. A study found that yoga can help stop the stress response in the hypothalamic part of the brain, which can provide relief for people with depression. In fact, the study found that yoga reduced cortisol levels better than antidepressants.

Practice Meditation

Research suggests that daily meditation isn't just feeling good right now - it can actually change the neural pathways in the brain, reducing anxiety and making you more resilient and stress-resistant. Never allow perceived ideas about which meditation should stop you from starting your routine. If you don't know meditation, you can start by following some guided meditations. You can access thousands of online meditation videos to help you get started.

Two types of meditations:

1. In concentration meditation, focus your consciousness on one point (for many people, it means repeating a short phrase, called a mantra).

2. In mindfulness meditation, allow various thoughts and sensations to roam the mind, examining them without judgment.

Both of these methods can be helpful in preparing the mind for intermittent fasting.

Meditation and deep breathing work together, but you can also quickly do deep breathing exercises alone, whenever you are experiencing increased stress or even when you don't feel it and want to stay ahead. When stressed, we breathe rapidly, take shallow breaths that come from our chest rather than your abdomen. When you breathe deeply from the abdomen, you absorb more oxygen, making you feel less anxious, less breathless, and more relaxed. Learning to breathe deeply requires practice, but the following steps will help you become a professional in deep breathing:

1. Sit upright or lie on your in an agreeable spot.

2. Breathe in profoundly through your nose. You should feel the hand on the midsection rise; however, the hand on the chest should move practically nothing.

3. Breathe out through your mouth, breathing out however much air as could be expected.

4. Rehash this procedure until you feel your body start to unwind. Listening to Music

Do you know that feeling when your favorite song plays, and you start singing, and you feel better immediately? There is a science behind it all. Research shows that whatever your mood is, listening to the music you love can lower cortisol levels. While any music you like can have an anti-stress effect, classical music works very well. Listening to classical music can reduce stress hormones, lower blood pressure, and reduce pulse and heart rate.

Notwithstanding physical impacts, music likewise redirects your consideration. Rather than becoming involved with your considerations or visiting consistently, the music ingests your consideration and powers you to concentrate on something different. Whenever you feel focused on, play old-style music or a tune you like. Rests and tune in or even move.

Keep a Diary

Writing your contemplations and dissatisfactions down has a demonstrated beneficial outcome on feelings of anxiety. You can likewise utilize your diary to make day by day thank you records. Recording only three things you're appreciative of consistently will assist you with promoting decrease worry by recalling the positive parts of your life. They don't need to be huge things. Indeed, checking out the seemingly insignificant details throughout your life will assist you with facilitating value your day by day encounters. You can compose things like "I'm appreciative to rest in a bed, or I'm thankful for some espresso." Try to pick various things consistently and you will perceive how appreciative you truly should be, in any event, for things you might not have given a lot of consideration to previously.

Keeping a journal is also useful for keeping track of your emotions and how those emotions affect your eating habits. Write down how you feel every day and what you eat. When you look back, you will be able to recognize how your emotions relate to food (the amount and types of food you eat) and focus on eliminating negative behaviors that you may not have. I have not been aware of the opposite.

Draw Strength from Your Friends

Studies show that nearby human bonds are basic for physical and emotional wellness and that social segregation can prompt expanded cortisol levels. The human touch animates the vagus nerve (one of the nerves that associates the cerebrum to the body), loosens up the sensory system, and stops the reaction to stretch. Contact additionally builds the arrival of oxytocin (a hormone identified with sentiments of unwinding, certainty, and mental strength), once in a while called love hormone, and lessens the arrival of cortisol.

Direct contact is the best solution, so find as much time as possible to communicate with your loved ones. Surround yourself with people who support you and who want to see you achieve your goals; Avoid combative or hostile people. Tense relationships can increase cortisol levels.

Make Your Life Easier in Your Fast

Just a starter of intermittent fasting or having a habit of eating five or six small meals or constantly grazing during the day, it can be a great transition to jump straight into fasting. It is not necessary to make a complete change overnight; in fact, you may be more successful if you get used to it slowly.

Start by moving from five or six small meals throughout the day to three regular-sized meals at a set time. You don't have to eat for a certain period of time yet; Get your body used to the habit and structure of the three-meal program. This will also require removing snacks throughout the day. Snacks are not prohibited when performing intermittent fasting, but it may be helpful to remove snacks during the early stages of adaptation.

Choose a Skip Meal

Once you are in the habit of a three-meal plan, choose a missed meal, and make a commitment to skip it every day for a few weeks. Don't spend too much time thinking about skipping meals; you can change your meal later if it fits your schedule or better. The goal is to get the body used to be without food for a long period of time. Sometimes the hardest part of fasting is getting your mind to accept the idea of skipping meals, which will get you used to the idea.

Reach Your Goal

When you start skipping meals and choosing the diet to follow, work slowly towards the ultimate goal of fasting. For example, if you follow the 16/8 method and have decided that the feeding period will be between 11 a.m. and at 7 p.m., but start by pushing the breakfast at 8:30 for a few days. So when you're used to having breakfast late, go back another hour and then another hour in a few days until your body feels comfortable waiting for 11 am in the morning to eat. Gradually postponing meals will not only help you relax mentally; it can also help you prevent or relieve some of the initial physical symptoms that may occur at the beginning of the intermittent fast.

Calculate Your Nutrition Plan

The next steps are to determine the type of diet you will follow and find delicious new recipes to incorporate into your plan. Complicated and refined recipes are always tempting and can be a weekend pleasure, but in the early stages of your new fasting plan, it will be easier to simplify things.

When you've just started turning on and off quickly, it's also helpful to cut down on your training routine. At the beginning of the fast, you may not have energy and motivation. This is completely normal. Instead of doing high-intensity exercises, keep your workouts light. You can resume your training routine in a few weeks when your body has adapted.

CHAPTER TWO- Understanding Fasting

Intermittent fasting means changing your attention on the body: what you put in it and what you think about it. Mental discipline is being developed to follow a new lifestyle and change, often dramatically, the way we think about what we eat and drink. The better you understand what fasting is, the more benefits you will get. Here, let's consider some of the things you can predict when you start intermittent fasting.

Prepare your Mind

As with any lifestyle change, intermittent fasting can be difficult at first. You may feel irritable or have little energy. You may be very hungry and have difficulty meeting your plan. Or you can feel good from the start, immediately get positive results, and feel empowered and motivated by your new lifestyle. It depends on your body. However, some things are likely to happen as you adjust to the new routine. When you know what to expect and have the tools ready to face the challenges that may arise, your chances of long-term success are much greater.

Consider these popular quotes: your mind will stop a thousand times before your body and your body can handle almost anything. It is your mind that you have to convince. The general message behind these two powerful sayings is that often when you surrender, it is not because you have reached your physical limit.

Find Mental Clarity

After completing the initial stages of intermittent fasting, you will likely notice important changes. Not only will your negative speech and your inclination to negativity decrease, but you will also experience greater mental clarity. Intermittent fasting tends to eliminate fog from the brain and facilitates focus. You may also experience a less simian mind: intrusive and quick thoughts that distract you from the task at hand and affect your productivity. You may notice that your productivity and energy level are increasing. Your memory may seem clearer,, and it may be easier for you to keep the new information than before. You may also notice a stabilization of your moods and emotions, even less anxiety,, and a happier temperament.

Yes, you will be Hungry!

It is impossible to say exactly how your body will feel during the early stages of intermittent fasting because each person is different, and you can react differently to others. However, there are some things that often happen to most people at the beginning of an intermittent fast. If you are used to eating five or six times a day, you may experience these effects more than if you already eat three meals a day with a minimum of snacks.

As your body adapts to intermittent fasting, it is normal to experience an increase in hunger and food cravings. It is often mental or emotional hunger rather than physical hunger. You may also experience headaches, lack of energy, and irritability. You may feel slightly dizzy, weak, or dizzy when you get up.

Your Body will stabilize!

After the initial rehabilitation period, your blood sugar and insulin levels begin to stabilize, and you will begin to enjoy the benefits of intermittent fasting. One of the first things you will probably notice is an increase in energy. You can feel sustained energy all day long; Instead of feeling awake and productive in the morning, but being hit by the terrible afternoon slump around 14:00 or 15:00, you will feel constant energy. This is explained by the fact that the blood sugar level does not increase and does not decrease as when eating several meals over the course of an entire day.

Say Goodbye to Swelling!

You may experience a reduction in inflammation, so any swelling on the face, skin, hands, or feet can begin to decrease. The chronic pain that is an integral part of your day can decrease or disappear completely. So, you may start to notice that you are losing a few extra pounds, falling asleep easier and that your sleep quality is better. You will move and turn less at night, and consequently, you will wake up rested and rested instead of being dazed and disoriented. If you exercise regularly, it may also be easier for you to complete your workouts.

Psychology of Hunger

Hunger is delicate because, on the one hand, there is a real physiological hunger; On the other hand, there is mental hunger. Simply put, physical hunger occurs when the stomach is empty. You may feel a physical emptiness in the stomach, as well as weakness or a drop in energy. Although you can do these things unconsciously, when you become aware of them, you can change the way they influence you. Instead of eating without thinking because you are participating in a social activity or because your partner is hungry, pay attention to what you really feel. Are you really hungry, or are you tempted by one of these clues? In the latter case, you can change your environment or use one of the few useful techniques provided in this chapter to reduce hunger.

Write It Down

A good way to track changes is to write down all the symptoms that occur before starting the intermittent fasting plan. Try to dig deeper and be really complete, even by listing the things you've been dealing with for a long time or that you think have nothing to do with your eating habits. After fasting for a few weeks, rewrite your list, and compare the two lists. Rewrite your list every two weeks thereafter. This can help you keep track of the improvements you may not even expect, and you will probably be pleasantly surprised.

Traces of Hunger

The signs of hunger make us eat, even when we are not hungry. There are three types of hunger indices: sensory, social, and regulatory.

An external sensory signal is all that arouses your desire to eat by focusing your senses. For example, you can smell your favorite food or see a container full of freshly baked cookies. Research shows that exposure to external sensory signals can significantly increase your desire to eat, even when your stomach is full, and you are not really hungry.

Food has become a way of entertaining people and pleasing others. Eating out now is a favorite pastime, and you can rarely go to a party or other event without being offered any type of food. These temptations are social clues. In many of these cases, you are likely to eat even if you are not hungry; often, you won't even notice it.

The last type of hunger index is the normative index; These are things like the portion or size of the dish that affects the amount of food you eat. You may not even realize that these things influence you, but research shows that when you use larger dishes, you tend to eat more and therefore eat more.

Drink Lots of Water

During fasting periods (and in general), water should be your best friend. You have probably heard that thirst is often confused with hunger, so staying hydrated can help reduce any false signs of hunger. When you wake up, drink a quarter of a liter of water. You can prepare yourself by drinking a glass of water on the bedside table when you go to sleep. Drink water regularly throughout the day. If you train a lot or lose a lot of sweat in some other way, you may have to drink more. You'll also need to add an additional glass of water to each cup of coffee or other diuretics you drink, so keep that in mind. The more hydrated you are, the less false signs of hunger you will have.

Reduce Stress

Stress is a big problem worldwide. About 77% of Americans report that they regularly experience physical symptoms of stress, and 33% of them report living in extreme stress. Stress can cause not only weight gain but also heart disease, diabetes, headache, depression, anxiety, and gastrointestinal problems. One of the immediate ways in which stress contributes to weight gain is by encouraging him to eat comfort foods, such as pizza or ice cream, which he may not want when his stress levels are better controlled. You have probably heard of emotional food. To avoid the dangers of stress, we recommend that you find ways to manage it. Stress management is particularly useful for avoiding hunger signals. Once the stress level is under control, you can focus your attention on your food plan and follow the steps that will help you achieve your goals.

Get Enough Sleep

The importance of sleep cannot be overstated, not only for preventing hunger but also for general health. Sleep is nourishing and regenerating, and when you don't have enough, it can completely destabilize you. When you're stressed out, it's easy to skimp on sleep and try removing some things from your to-do list, but don't do it! Sleep time is the time when the brain and body repair and recharge, and it is essential to control stress levels and hunger hormones. Sleep also helps improve mood and energy levels, increases concentration, and willpower, which is extremely important in the early stages of intermittent fasting.

Stay Focused

The most important thing you can do to ensure your success with intermittent fasting is to have a plan. The first step is to determine what type of fasting you are going to do. After determining the type of fast, establish a schedule. Are you going to fast every day? At what time will you fast, and at what time do you feed? Once the timeline is established, another essential element is determining what you will eat when you enter your food state. Will you follow a specific diet (like the keto diet or the Paleo diet), or will you follow a clean basic diet without real rules?

Design your Food Plan

You will first need to develop your eating plan. You can plan a few days, a week, or even the whole month. Find simple recipes and write down everything you eat and at what time. When you start with intermittent fasting and meal planning, excitement can lead you to seek imagination, new recipes or a lot of variety, but when you are in the early stages of a new lifestyle, one of the most beneficial things you can do is stick to the bases, not making it too complicated.

Follow What You Know

Stick to the foods you already know and recipes that don't take long to prepare or that require you to learn new cooking skills or purchase new kitchen utensils. You will have plenty of time to try new things after getting used to the basics, and your body and mind will adapt to the changes. The goal of preparing meals is to make you feel less overwhelmed, not to add unnecessary stress.

There are online meal planners and trackers, as well as telephone apps that you can use to track your meals, but you don't need fancy tools or software if the technology isn't available. You can simplify it by recording everything in a notebook.

Create a Shopping List

After preparing your recipes and your food plan, it's time to find out what you need. Check your fridge and pantry before writing your shopping list, so you don't buy what you already have. After making a list of the things you have at hand, make a shopping list of the other items you will need to prepare for your recipes and meals for the week (or for the period of time you choose).

You can save even more time by organizing your shopping list based on the location of the items in the supermarket. You can list all chilled meats, products, and items together. If you have to go to different stores for any offer or specialized item, organize your lists by the shop.

Prepare Your Meals

After learning the basics, preparing meals can help you stay on track and prevent you from eating an unhealthy meal when you are hungry. Research shows that people who prepare meals early are more successful in achieving their health and nutrition goals and save time and money in the long run. As you enter the rhythm of intermittent fasting and your new way of eating, you can adjust your meals and your preparation routine.

The organization is one of the most important elements for good meal preparation. It may seem intimidating or wastes of time to sit, organize recipes, and write everything, but it will save you time.

How much you prepare in advance and how much time you spend cooking depends entirely on you. Some people spend three to four hours on Sundays, preparing meals for the whole week. Others spend a few hours on Sundays preparing meals for the next few days, then spend a few more hours preparing meals for the rest of the week. Whatever style of food preparation you choose, an organization is essential.

Before and After

Instead, take photos sooner or later (or progress). In the end, you can compare them side by side to see how your body has changed over time. Photos can be a very motivating tool because when you see yourself every day, you may not notice the small changes that are happening, but when you compare photos that were taken a month later, the changes can be much more noticeable. Don't let your body's current dissatisfaction stop you from taking photos first. You will be happy to have them on the road.

Body Measurements

It is helpful to take body measurements. You can start developing leaner muscle mass, especially if you exercise or weight regularly. When your body starts to change, you may not notice too many changes on the scale, but your body composition can change radically. Measurements can help you track your progress by documenting missing thumbs on different parts of your body.

What to Measure:

You will need to follow the following steps:

Bust: measure the entire bust, keeping the tape measure in line with your nipples.

Chest: measure directly under the breast or pectoral muscles and around the back.

Hips: find the widest part of the hips and measure around it.

Knees: measure around the knee, directly above the knee, standing.

Forearm: measure around the widest part of the forearm under the elbow.

Thighs: Measure around the fullest part of the leg while standing.

Arm: measure around the widest part of the arm above the elbow.

Waist: Find the narrowest part of the waist, usually just below the rib cage, and measure around it.

To measure correctly, you need a non-extensible tape measure. When taking measurements, wrap the tape around the body as close to the skin as possible, but do not over tighten it so that the tape measure does not cut or dent the skin. It helps if someone else takes your measurements for you so that you can stand up straight; If you don't have anyone available, take your measurements in front of a mirror to make sure you keep the tape level and measure in the right places.

There will be Ups and Downs

Like everything in life, you will experience ups and downs with intermittent fasting, especially in the beginning. Don't expect everything to work from the beginning, and don't let yourself be captivated by perfection. You're about to make a mistake: sometimes you will eat outside of your feeding period, and that's fine. If you go there knowing that you will do your best, but also understand that it may take some time to get used to the transition, you will be less likely to get hurt when things don't go as planned.

CHAPTER THREE- Fasting and Healthy Lifestyle

One of the most common reasons why people participate in intermittent fasting is weight loss, but this only scratches the surface. Intermittent fasting does a lot more for your body than helping you lose weight. It also helps stabilize blood sugar, reduces chronic or diffuse inflammation, and improves your heart health. Studies have also shown that intermittent fasting can contribute to brain health and help reduce the risk of developing serious brain diseases such as Alzheimer's disease. Finally, some researchers have suggested that it can help prevent cancer and improve the effects of chemotherapy in people with the disease.

Intermittent Fasting and Diets

Studies also show that people who follow diets that allow for variability in food choices, such as intermittent fasting, are more likely to follow their diet and maintain weight loss than those on a diet. Rigid and calorie-controlled diet. Stiff diets are also associated with symptoms of eating disorders and a higher body mass index (a measure of body fat based on weight and height) in non-obese women, while flexible dieting strategies such as intermittent fasting are not.

Hearing this can be overwhelming, particularly in the event that you have bought into the hypothesis that the best approach to get thinner is to cut calories and train more, yet it's, in reality, uplifting news. You don't need to go through your days checking calories, eating nearly nothing, and keeping away from solid fats. There is a superior way: irregular fasting. (Only a note here: fasting functions admirably for certain individuals and not others. You need to locate the ideal approach to shed pounds, the one that works best for you.)

Women and Fasting

In general, fasting is believed to be harmful to women, and although this may be true of some women, it is not a general claim that can be applied to all women. This theory has been developed due to the fact that intermittent fasting has the potential to cause hormonal imbalance in some women if fasting is not performed correctly, but when proper precautions and care are taken, women can successfully fast.

Since the female body was physiologically designed to carry children, women are more sensitive to hunger than men. If a woman's body feels imminent hunger, she will respond by increasing the hormones leptin and ghrelin, which work together to control hunger. This hormonal response is the way the female body protects the developing fetus, even if the woman is not currently pregnant.

While the signs of hunger in ghrelin and leptin can be ignored, it becomes increasingly difficult, especially when the body rebels and starts producing more of these hormones. On the off chance that a lady is eager in an undesirable manner, eating or eating unfortunate nourishments can cause a course of other hormonal issues identified with insulin.

This procedure can likewise close down the conceptive framework. In the event that your body figures, it needs more food to endure, it could stop your capacity to imagine to secure a potential pregnancy. That is the reason fasting isn't suggested during pregnancy or for ladies attempting to get pregnant.

Intermittent and Your Body Type

Fasting and Autophagy

Self-healing is a normal physiological process that involves removing ancient or destructive compounds from the body while this seems a little worrying; the literal translation of autophagy is being devoured. It comes from the Greek machines, which translate into yourself and false, which means to eat. The term autophagy was coined by the Nobel Prize-winning scientist Christian de Duve after a team of researchers noted an increase in lysosomes (parts of the cells responsible for breaking down and destroying other compounds) in the liver cells after the injection of glucagon, the hormone that acts against insulin.

Autophagy assumes a key job in looking after homeostasis, a steady and sound interior condition in the body. Your body continually contains proteins and organelles (particular little structures in every one of your body's cells) that become useless or die. Whenever permitted to amass in the body, these dead tissues can cause cell demise, add to tissue and organ breakdown, and even become harmful. During autophagy, the body marks harmed portions of cells and unused proteins in the body. These harmed parts are sent to the lysosomes, where they are expelled from the body. This procedure keeps them from causing hurt.

Method 16/8

When following the 16/8 method, plan a 16-hour fasting period and an eight-hour feeding period each day. This means that you will spend sixteen hours eating nothing and that you will eat all your meals in eight consecutive hours. For example, you can choose a quick window between 7 p.m. and 11 in the morning, which means that the power window is between 11 in the morning and 7 p.m.

Drinking While Fasting

During the fasting period, you can drink water, coffee and other non-caloric drinks, such as tea or mineral water;

however, watch your caffeine intake and be careful not to overdo it. While drinking drinks during the fasting period can help prevent hunger, too much caffeine can cause anxiety, nerves and dehydration, especially when the stomach is empty. Caffeine also exerts pressure on the adrenal glands, therefore, since the body adapts to the additional stress of fasting, it is better to minimize coffee intake.

One of the main advantages of the 16/8 intermittent fasting method is that it is quite easy to integrate into your schedule. Since you will sleep for about eight hours after your fast, you will only have to skip food for a small part of your waking hours. Most people can be successful with the 16/8 method by not eating after dinner and then skipping breakfast or eating it late in the morning.

Eat Raw Foods

While there is no specific diet to follow when performing the 16/8 method, Martin Berkhan, who developed the method, recommends that whole and unprocessed foods make up the majority of the calorie intake. You may need to monitor sales carefully and buy in bulk, but unprocessed foods may fit into your meal budget. It just takes a bit of arranging. Notwithstanding eating as neatly as could be expected under the circumstances, you have to consolidate protein into a moderate segment of your calorie admission. When you work out, the greater part of the calories you don't get from protein should originate from starches. On rest days, fat admission ought to be more prominent than starch consumption.

The Warrior Diet

The warrior diet, which was created by Ori Hofmekler, an individual from the Israeli Special Forces, is viewed as the impetus for other intermittent fasting strategies. Hofmekler presented the warrior diet in 2001 in the wake of investing energy in the military and examining the conduct and dietary patterns of the war social orders of Rome and Sparta. He structured the warriors' eating regimen dependent on the conviction that it was the normal method to eat before the modern transformation and that, tailing it; it could advance both weight reduction and an expansion in vitality.

The warrior regime pushes the 16/8 method a little further by extending the fasting period to almost twenty hours. While following the warrior's diet, you only eat one large meal at night. During the day, you can have light snacks, such as berries, yogurt and whey protein, as well as water, vegetable juices, coffee and tea. The fasting part of the warrior's diet is the under-meal phase and the four-hour feeding window is the overeating phase.

The malnutrition phase occurs during the day because the stress of less food triggers the fight or flight response of the sympathetic nervous system. Therefore, there is an expansion in vitality, an increment in adrenaline (which advances

49

sharpness) and an expansion in fat consuming. The gorging stage happens around evening time in light of the fact that the objective during this stage is to do something contrary to the non-eating stage by activating rest and stomach related reaction of the parasympathetic sensory system. At the point when the body is in rest and processing mode, it advances quiet and unwinding, improves absorption and enables the body to recoup from the pressure of the day. When the body is relaxed, it can also use the nutrients it absorbs more efficiently.

Limitations on Food Pairings

In contrast to other fasting methods, which don't determine precisely what kinds of food to eat during the fasting time frame, the warrior's eating regimen limits certain mixes of nourishments. For instance, while following the warrior's eating regimen, you can consolidate proteins and vegetables; however you ought to abstain from joining nuts, products of the soil, proteins and oats, liquor and starch. The hypothesis behind this is your body can process some food blends superior to other people. The blend of proteins and vegetables helps assimilation, while the mix of proteins and grains makes processing troublesome.

During the four-hour time frame that you will eat, you will begin eating vegetables, proteins and non-dull fats. Once introduced, you can include sugars in case you're as yet ravenous. The hypothesis behind this is eating thusly can upgrade hormone creation and how the body consumes fat for the duration of the day.

Nonetheless, the warrior's eating routine doesn't concentrate just on intermittent fasting; The genuine warrior diet additionally requires normal exercise during fasting. As per examine, you can wreck to 20% progressively fat when turning out to be on an unfilled stomach. The hypothesis is that high insulin levels can smother the manner in which the body uses fat. When fasting, insulin levels decline. In the event that you initiate your digestion by practicing when insulin levels are low, you can consume increasingly fat.

The Eat Stop Eat Method

Rather than fasting each day, the Eat Stop Eat method comprises of consolidating a 24-hour quick for a couple of days seven days, at that point eating the other five or six days ordinarily. With the Eat Stop Eat method, pick the days and times of your quick, yet you should make a point not to eat for 24 hours. For instance, your timetable may expend ordinarily from Tuesday to Sunday, yet fasting from Sunday evening at 8pm. until Monday at 20:00 As with the 16/8 method, you can't eat food during fasting periods, yet you can drink without calorie drinks. At the point when the quick finishes, begin eating again ordinarily.

Brad Pilon, originator of the Eat Stop Eat method, accepts that you are educated to eat since the beginning at specific occasions, and this thought can test you and test you on how you by and large feel. He characterizes intermittent fasting as the capacity to rehearse persistence with regards to eating - cognizant and gracious balance with regards to eating. Their way of thinking is that we don't have to eat constantly, so we are allowed to pick when we eat.

Since the Eat Stop Eat method focuses primarily on meals, Pilon does not define foods as prohibited or prohibited. You don't need to count calories or limit your diet, and not doing one or another makes monitoring your feeding days easier, but if you want optimal results or if your goal is to lose weight, you will have to make wise decisions when it comes to diet.

The 5:2 Method

The 5: 2 Method, additionally called the quick and quick 5:2 eating regimen, was promoted by Michael Mosley, a British specialist and columnist. The 5:2 methods include fasting just on specific days of the week. With this fasting method, you will never totally cease from eating: you as a rule eat five days every week, and afterward limit the calories to 500-600 calories for each day on the other two days of the week.

If follow the 5:2 methods, you can eat regularly on Monday, Wednesday, Thursday, Saturday and Sunday, yet limit the calories on Tuesday and Friday. Pick the times of the week you quick, however you have to incorporate a non-quick day among your quick days.

The typical eating routine relies upon tallness, weight, sex, level of physical movement and weight objectives. There are a few free online number crunchers (you can look through the online calorie adding machine to discover numerous choices) that permit you to enter insights and objectives and get a proposal on what number of calories you ought to devour during your ordinary days.

Alternate-Day Fasting

There are two forms of alternative fasting. The first, and less common, is to alternate between days of normal fasting and days of complete fasting. This means that you would normally eat on Monday, you will completely refrain from eating on Tuesday, you will normally eat on Wednesday, and you will completely keep from Thursday, and so on. The second way is to change the fast. When he alternately follows the modified fast, he eats normally on alternate days and consumes about a fifth of his normal calories on the remaining days. For a typical diet of 2,000 to 2,500 calories per day, that means you would eat 400 to 500 calories during your fast modified days. The goal is to cut calories from 20 to 35% per week. Research shows that people can follow a fast alternation of a day much easier than traditional low-calorie diets that require a calorie restriction every day of the week.

Like many other fasting methods, you can drink as many calorie-free drinks as you want while fasting. If you choose to follow the modified version of the fast, there are no restrictions on the consumption of calories during the day. You can have a big meal during the day or distribute mini-meals or snacks during the day.

Spontaneous Fasting

Unlike other types of fasting, which are more rigid in their specific duration, spontaneous fasting involves the spontaneous skipping of meals. For example, if you are not hungry in the morning, skip lunch and eat only lunch and dinner. Or if you're too busy for lunch, skip it.

However, the key to spontaneous fasting is to make sure you are eating healthy foods for meals that don't skip. Of course, this is important for all types of fasting, but it can be especially important for spontaneous fasting, as there is less structure and the temptation to eat too much unhealthy food can be stronger.

Extended Fasting

Although extended fasting falls into a separate category, it is important to know the difference between prolonged fasting and other types of intermittent fasting. Prolonged fasting is any type of fasting that lasts more than twenty-four hours.

Prolonged fasting can often last for a week, and many of these prolonged fasting only concern drinking water.

These types of fasting are most common in the medical and hospital setting and are generally performed when the body is about to recover significantly or when the ability to eat is impaired. Prolonged fasting should not be initiated without the recommendation and supervision of a health professional.

Choosing the Best Plan for You

There are many variations of intermittent fasting because there is no one size suitable for all approaches. Plans work differently; one that works best for your neighbor may not work for you and vice versa. To decide which type of intermittent fasting is best for you, you should ask yourself a series of questions.

One of the most important things you should do is determine which type of diet is best for your program. Sure, it's possible to rearrange your schedule based on your new eating plan and for some people it may be necessary, but it's more likely that you will stick to a new routine if it gets a little easy your Life. The 16/8 method is the best plan for their program because fasting is most often done at night. However, if you don't have a regular work schedule or if your working hours are longer and you have to stay for a longer part of the day, this may not work as well for you. For example, if you don't work normally from

Monday to Friday and have a Monday and Thursday off, you may find that the 5: 2 methods works best for your schedule because you can eat normally while at work and then use your days off for your fasting days.

What Plan Will you Follow?

Sometimes it's not enough to know which plan best fits your schedule. To get the long-term benefits of intermittent fasting, you need to stick to it. You will need to find a plan suitable for your program. If the 16/8 method seems the best in theory, but you know that you would have problems staying sixteen hours without food, then perhaps a modified protocol for another day's fast would be better for you.

Don't push yourself too hard to be perfect or to follow a certain protocol to the letter, especially at the beginning. Adapting to intermittent fasting can take some time, especially if you are used to eating small meals throughout the day. Be kind to yourself and take the time to adapt and adapt.

Mix and Match

You can utilize the methods portrayed to create your convention or you can likewise blend the conventions as you go. For instance, you can follow the nuts and bolts of the 16/8 method, yet rapidly for thirteen or fourteen hours rather than sixteen. You can utilize Eat Stop Eat as a model, however quick from sixteen to eighteen hours for a couple of days every week until you can proceed onward to a twenty-four hour quick. Keep in mind, the best way to make the two methods work is in the event that you can tail it. Transforming one of the conventions for long haul consistence is better than attempting to follow a convention precisely as it is composed and leaving it following half a month since you are disappointed.

Exercise during Fasting.

There is a last discussion in the wellness world about whether it is smarter to prepare on a vacant stomach (a fasting state) or an entire one (a fed state). The appropriate response is that it relies upon the power of the activity. Practicing on a vacant stomach has numerous advantages, yet in the event that you are a perseverance competitor or are doing a high force work out, practicing after a supper might be best for you.

When you train, your body needs more energy. First, your body will convert the fuel into blood glucose. When it runs out, it starts burning glycogen, the form of glucose stored in the liver. In general, the liver stores enough glycogen to meet the body's energy needs for 24 hours without food; however, the increased demand for energy that exercise exerts on the body will lead to a faster reduction in glycogen. The amount of glycogen used depends on the duration and intensity of the exercise you do.

Once the glycogen is depleted, your body switches from carbohydrates that burn for energy to stored fats. The body's ability to burn fat is controlled by the sympathetic nervous system, which is activated by fasting and exercise. When the two are combined, the physiological processes that split fat into energy are maximized. Unlike glycogen, which is an only stored in limited quantity, fats can be stored in your body in unlimited quantities, so they will never run out. Your muscles will eventually adapt to any energy source you give them.

The Hormonal Benefits of Fasting Exercise

In addition to increasing fat burning, fasting exercise has also been shown to improve health by improving the levels of two specific hormones: insulin and growth hormone.

Research shows that fasting exercise can have a positive effect on insulin sensitivity (the way the body reacts to insulin). When you overeat, your blood sugar levels skyrocket, and as a result, your body is exposed to a constant flow of insulin. Over time, this can cause insulin overload which weakens the way the cells respond to the hormone. Practicing on a empty stomach not just keeps the body from discharging insulin into the blood, it additionally copies any overabundance insulin that you may have. At the point when your body reacts to insulin in a solid manner, it is simpler to lose fat and improve blood flow to the muscles, which enables work to muscle. Fasting exercise expands development hormone creation, which consumes fat and builds muscle tissue, yet additionally improves bone wellbeing.

High Intensity Exercise

The days you want to do high intensity exercise, such as high intensity training (HIIT), a type of workout where you will alternate short periods of high intensity exercise with longer periods of low intensity exercise or weight training. Come on; plan your workout near a meal. When you train in a nutritious state, you are supplying your body with glucose and glycogen to help you do your workouts. This will prevent muscle loss and hypoglycaemia.

A good way to measure your training intensity is the voice test. During a low intensity workout, you should be able to continue a conversation easily enough. When the exercise is very intense, you should be able to speak only a few words comfortably at a time. If you can't speak during training without losing your breath, you train too much.

Exercise Tips

Regular training is an essential part of staying healthy, so while little additional planning is needed to get the right pace when you fast intermittently, it is important to maintain a regular routine. Always listen to the specific needs of his body again.

On the off chance that you are hoping to manufacture genuine muscle, plan all quality preparing between suppers. Your muscles need amino acids to fix and develop after weight lifting, so in the event that you need to include muscle, eat a high protein supper one hour before muscle preparing and another high protein dinner. 60 to an hour and a half subsequent to preparing. As per the Academy of Nutrition and Dietetics, 20-30 grams of top notch protein per supper ought to be focused on.

Remember that numerous individuals effectively eat considerably more than the suggested protein necessity consistently, so you don't need to go insane. To give you somewhat viewpoint, a 170 g chicken breast contains 52 grams of protein.

CHAPTER FOUR- Ingredients for a Healthy Fasting Diet

The intermittent fasting lifestyle does not simply mean not eating; it's also about being more aware of the food you eat. Just as there are various fasting methods, there are several diets that you can follow, including Paleo, Low Carb and Paste. You have to find what works for you and get what you want. In addition, good decisions must be made when buying food, finding food and drinks that promote maximum health.

Maintain a relationship of carbohydrates, proteins and fats.

The most important diets emphasize macronutrients (carbohydrates, proteins and fats). There are low carbohydrate, fat and fat and carbohydrate diets. There is also IIFYM, "if it fits your macros", which is based on the principle that you can eat what you want as long as it maintains the right carbohydrate, protein and fat ratio for your body. Although some of these diets focus on food quality, many of them lack an important piece of the health puzzle: micronutrients. Carbohydrates, proteins and fats are macronutrients; Vitamins and minerals are micronutrients. However, just because the body needs smaller amounts of micronutrients doesn't mean they are less important. Indeed, the importance of obtaining adequate quantities of micronutrients cannot be overstated.

The Importance of Micronutrients

Thirteen vitamins and sixteen minerals (called micronutrients) are needed in adequate quantities every day. These vitamins and minerals help to maintain all bodily functions in the right way. Some affect your blood; others help you metabolize carbohydrates, proteins and fats. Of course, this only touches the surface. These and other vitamins and minerals play many other roles in your body.

If your intake of vitamins and minerals is reduced, you will eventually develop a deficiency. Although it may not seem like a big deal, even a small deficiency of a micronutrient can cause serious health problems. Low levels of vitamin D have been associated with depression (particularly seasonal affective disorder, which occurs in the winter months) and irritable bowel syndrome. Magnesium deficiency can cause irregular heartbeat, muscle spasms and cramps, hypertension, fatigue, depression and apathy (lack of emotion). Vitamin B12 deficiencies can present psychological conditions, such as dementia, paranoia and major depression.

The Ketogenic Diet

The ketogenic diet is one of the most popular diet companions for intermittent fasting. People who love intermittent fasting tend to follow this diet because the two approaches complement each other so well: if used in combination, they will quickly lead to a chronic state of ketosis (a physiological state in which your body burns fat for energy from carbohydrates).

Following a keto diet, most of the calories come from fat and carbohydrate intake will be severely limited. Unlike other diets, a keto diet requires you to track the exact amount of fat, carbohydrates and proteins you are eating.

A typical ketogenic diet has a breakdown of macronutrients as follows:

- 60 to 75 percent of calories from fat
- 15-30 percent of calories from protein
- 5-10 percent of calories from carbohydrates

The Paleo Diet

The Paleo diet is another popular intermittent fasting companion because, like fasting, it is designed by the eating habits of your ancestors. The basic concept of a Paleo diet is to consume only foods available for hunters and gatherers during the Paleolithic era. Of course, this definition is open to interpretation because your Paleolithic ancestors would not have access to things like almond butter jars, but the idea is understood.

By following a Paleo diet, you can eat:

- Eggs
- Fish
- Fruits

- Healthy fats (avocado oil, coconut oil, olive oil, butter)
- Meat
- Natural sweeteners (raw honey, maple syrup, coconut sugar)
- Walnuts and seeds
- Poultry

On the other hand, you should avoid:

- Alcohol
- Dairy products (milk, cheese, ice cream, butter)
- Grains (wheat, oats, barley, rye, quinoa, couscous, amaranth, millet, corn)
- Legumes (soy, peanuts, chickpeas, beans)
- Refined and artificial sweeteners (white sugar, high fructose corn syrup, sucralose, and aspartame)

The Pegan Diet

Diet sticks are a fairly new concept developed by Dr. Mark Hyman, director of the Cleveland Clinical Center for Functional Medicine. The Pegan diet combines the basic principles of the Paleo diet and a vegan diet, which seems contradictory since at first glance the diets seem to be completely opposite to the spectrum; however, its basic principles are actually very similar.

Both the Paleo diet and the vegan diet emphasize the choice of whole and unprocessed foods that responsibly come from the earth. The main difference are that the Paleo diet focuses on ethically sourced meats, vegetables, healthy fats and some fruits and eliminates all cereals and legumes; A vegan diet eliminates all animal products and emphasizes cereals, legumes, vegetables and all plant-based foods. The goal of the stick diet is to combine the better of the two diets.

What Can You Eat In the Diet Stick?

Following the dietetic stick, plant-based foods will account for about 75 percent of the daily intake. We advise you to eat mainly vegetables; some fruits; some gluten-free cereals, such as quinoa, brown rice and gluten-free oatmeal; and some legumes, such as lentils. The other 25% of food intake should be in the form of high-quality animal proteins (grass-fed beef, grazing chicken and eggs) and healthy fats such as coconut, olives and avocados (and their respective oils: coconut oil, olive oil and avocado oil). Dr. Hyman recommends treating the meat more as a seasoning than as a main course. Instead of a typical 4-6 ounce serving, keep with 2-3 ounces of meat per meal.

By following the sticky diet, you will avoid gluten, dairy products and some vegetable oils (rapeseed, sunflower, corn and soy). Sugar, even natural types like honey and maple syrup, should only be consumed as an occasional treatment. Although natural sugars offer some health benefits, overdoing it can negatively affect blood sugar levels, something that you are ultimately trying to avoid when intermittent fasting.

The Low FODMAP Diet

FODMAPs (fermentable oligosaccharides, disaccharides, monosaccharides and polyols) are short chain carbohydrates that can cause digestive problems in people with digestive sensitivity. A low FODMAP diet is generally recommended for those with chronic digestive problems or unexplained irritable bowel syndrome. By following a low FODMAP diet, you will avoid certain categories of carbohydrates, including:

- Oligosaccharides: wheat, rye, legumes, garlic, onion, leeks, asparagus, jicama, fennel, beetroot and Brussels sprouts.
- Disaccharides: white sugar, milk, yogurt and soft cheeses such as cream cheese and ricotta.
- Monosaccharaides: peaches, plums, pears, nectarines, mangoes, watermelons, apples and honey.
- Polyols: blackberries, avocados, sweet potatoes, cauliflower, peas and mushrooms.

By following a low FODMAP diet, you will completely eliminate all FODMAP-rich foods for about a month. After this initial elimination period, you can reintroduce one high FODMAP food at a time to see how your body reacts. If a digestive disorder does not occur, the body can probably handle that food. If you experience digestive disorders, you are likely to be sensitive to that food and would do well to avoid it as much as possible.

The Low Carbohydrate Diet

A low carbohydrate diet is similar to a ketogenic diet in that it limits the amount of carbohydrates you eat every day. However, a traditional low-carb diet is not as rich in fat and allows for a more moderate protein intake than a ketogenic diet. Many low carbohydrate diets suggest a very low initial carbohydrate intake period, about two weeks, in which almost all carbohydrate foods are eliminated, except for low carbohydrate vegetables. During this initial period, you will lose a significant amount of water weight. After these two weeks, you will move on to a more sustainable program where you can include healthy sources of carbohydrates, like other vegetables, some fruits and whole grains without gluten. The main goal of a standard low-carbohydrate diet is to reduce blood sugar and insulin levels and promote weight loss.

Wheat

Wheat has been part of agriculture for over nine thousand years and is one of the largest crops in the world. It is considered an integral part of the food supply of many nations because it can be stored for years in the form of wheat and can be processed to produce a wide variety of foods, including flour, bread, pasta and cereals. The problem with wheat is not in the wheat itself, but in what modern agriculture has done to it.

Today's wheat is not only lower in many nutrients than it used to be, but the structure of the plant itself has changed due to modern grinding. The goal of modern processes is to create a crop that can survive in the event of a disaster, which is why large food companies have made it resistant to drought, bad weather, pests and chemicals. As a result, your body doesn't recognize wheat as it once did. Instead of providing food, wheat has become inflammatory and addicting.

It seems that nutrition experts and the general population are split in half when it comes to figuring out whether the beans are good or bad for you. One part of the debate recommends avoiding cereals, while the other party says that whole grains are a must because of their fiber and vitamin B content. The anti-grain side says there are three main problems with cereals: lectins, phytates and gluten.

Lectins, proteins that bind to cell membranes, are found in both cereals and legumes. They are small and difficult to digest because they are resistant to both heat and digestive enzymes. For this reason, they tend to accumulate in your body and travel to your blood in all its forms. When proteins enter your whole blood, your immune system develops antibodies, which means that it recognizes the protein as a foreign invader and creates an attack system against it. Over time, this can result in a loss of bowel and increased sensitivity to lectins.

Phytates are compounds found mainly in cereals and legumes and in smaller quantities in nuts and seeds. Phytates are not intrinsically harmful to you, but are often described as antinutrients because they bind to minerals such as iron, zinc and calcium, preventing their absorption. This can prepare you for mineral deficiencies. It is important to note here that phytates do not compromise your ability to absorb long-term nutrients; they block absorption only during that meal.

Go Gluten Free

Of course, when it comes to cereals, gluten is the most controversial. While celiac disease, the inability to properly digest gluten, is widely accepted, many people do not believe in sensitivity to non-celiac gluten. But research shows that gluten can damage the intestinal lining (and cause celiac disease symptoms) even in people who don't have the disease. Gluten-free cereals include brown rice, wild rice, quinoa, buckwheat, millet, teff and amaranth. Oatmeal is also technically gluten-free, but due to the way it is made, it is almost always contaminated with gluten. If you want to include oatmeal in your diet, choose brands that are specifically labeled gluten-free.

Make Your Cereals Healthier

Soak the beans before consuming them. Soaking the beans can help break down the phytates and neutralize the lectins, making the beans easier to digest and absorbing all the minerals they contain. To dip the beans, put them in a bowl and cover them completely with warm, filtered water. For each cup of water you add to the bowl, you should also add a spoonful of acid medium, such as lemon juice or apple cider vinegar. For example, if you need 3 cups of water to cover your beans, add 3 tablespoons of lemon juice to the water, then cover the container with a breathable medium, such as a clean tea towel.

Then let the beans rest for twelve hours. After the beans have been soaked for an adequate period of time, rinse them in cold water and continue with the recipe as usual. Another option is to sprout your cereals or use cereals that have already sprouted. Food manufacturers have taken advantage of the health benefits of germinating cereals, and many companies now offer already sprouted cereals, which can save you time and effort. If you can't find cereals that have already sprouted in your local supermarket, you can search online or sprout them yourself.

Sprout Your Beans

Germination takes much longer than soaked grains because you have to wait for the grain actually to open and sprout. To germinate your beans, follow the soaking process and then transfer the soaked and drained beans to a glass jar; a Mason bottle works well. Cover the jar with cheesecloth and let the beans rest in the wet jar at room temperature for one or five days. You will know when they are ready because the beans will open and you will see a green sprout. You can store sprouted cereals in the refrigerator for up to a week.

Dairy

Milk is another controversial product in the world of nutrition. You probably grew up listening to how good milk is for your bones. The truth is, milk is not as good for your bones as you might think. Countries with the lowest milk consumption have the lowest fracture rates and osteoporosis, a condition in which bones become fragile and are more prone to fractures and fractures. Also, many people have difficulty digesting the proteins and sugars found in milk. This is because with age, the body's production of lactase, the enzyme it needs to digest milk properly, naturally decreases.

However, this does not mean that you cannot consume any dairy products, but there are some better options than others. If you plan to include dairy products in your diet, choose dairy products that come from grass-fed cows. Usually grass-fed milk, butter and cheese can be found in local stores. Grass-fed dairy products have higher omega-3 content, unlike conventional dairy products, which have more omega-6. Omega-6s are not intrinsically bad, but when you overeat (which many Americans do), it can lead to chronic inflammation. Herb-fed dairy products, such as yogurt and

71

kefir, are also good options; however, make sure they are fat and simple. Flavored yogurt and kefir are often loaded with sugar.

Go With the Goats

If you want to avoid cow's milk entirely, the goat dairy is an excellent choice. Modern cow's milk contains large quantities of a protein called beta-casein A1, which can be very inflammatory and cause problems like eczema and acne. On the other hand, goat milk contains a protein called beta-casein A2, which is not inflammatory. Studies show that people who consume beta-casein A2 milk have experienced reduced inflammation and no negative digestive symptoms.

Goat milk is also more environmentally responsible than cow milk, as goats consume less grass and take up less space than cows. The soil needed to support two cows can support six goats.

Meat and Poultry

Meat is another controversial product that has been vilified over the years for its saturated fat content. When low-fat diets became very popular, red meat was a big no-no; but since then, science has shown that saturated fat doesn't have as big an impact on heart disease as previously thought. In fact, the correct types of saturated fat can protect against heart disease.

The old school of thought was that saturated fat increased cholesterol, increasing the risk of heart disease; but research now shows that while saturated fat can increase the amount of LDL in the blood, it creates large, fluffy LDL particles that don't stick to the walls of the arteries (compared to small, dense LDL particles. They get trapped in the arterial walls and can cause blockages, increasing the risk of heart disease.) Saturated fat also increases HDL levels, which is what protects against heart disease.

Meat is also one of the main sources of vitamin B12. In fact, you can only get vitamin B12 from animal products (although it is added to some foods, including some fortified cereals). The meat also contains other B vitamins, vitamin D, vitamin E, amino acids, antioxidants and various minerals.

Choose Grass-Fed Meat

As with dairy products, it is important to choose high-quality grass-fed meats. Conventional meat comes from cows fed crops, cereals and even sugar (genetically modified organisms). This fattens cows faster, therefore produces more, but affects the nutritional content of their meat. Grass-fed meat contains up to five times more omega-3 fatty acids than conventional meat and significantly less omega-6.

Grass-fed meat also contains a fat called conjugated linoleic acid or CLA. CLA acts as an antioxidant and has been shown to reduce the risk of heart disease, stop the growth of cancerous tumors, prevent atherosclerosis, lower triglycerides and reduce the risk of developing type-2 diabetes. All foods of animal origin contain a certain amount of CLA, but grass-fed meat and dairy products contain up to 500 percent more than dairy products and dairy cow meat.

Poultry

As with meat, not all birds are created equal. There are poultry that come from conventional farms, and then there are poultry that is organically raised and left to roam freely, following a natural diet. You will often see labels on birds and eggs that boast that the birds have been "fed a vegetarian diet", but chickens and turkeys are not vegetarian. They like to hunt insects, ticks and worms, which is what makes their meat so nutritious. Poultry that have been allowed to consume a natural diet are richer in omega-3s, vitamins and minerals.

When choosing poultry, it is best to choose a combination of organic and herb products. If this isn't available in your local supermarket or your budget doesn't allow it, talk to your local farmers. Often on your local farms you can find high quality meats that are not labeled as pasture or organic (because these are moderate terms by the government and many small farms cannot afford the certification process required to carry the labels), but for definition are both.

Eggs

There is a lot of fear around cholesterol, so people often separate their eggs, throw the yolk away and eat only the egg white. While egg white contains proteins, most of the nutrients, such as vitamins A, D, E and K; Omega-3 fats of B vitamins; football; and phosphorus are found in its bud. Don't be afraid to eat the whole egg, but choose the types of eggs you eat wisely.

Many of the nutrition labels and egg claims are just marketing tactics. For example, the terms natural and farm-fresh generally mean nothing. Other terms, like cageless, sound good, but they can be misleading. When you hear the term cage-free, you can imagine birds roaming outside in the sunlight, but without a cage it just means that the birds weren't caged. They could still have been in a crowded warehouse without much room to move. The best types of eggs you can get are organic and grazing. Again, talking to local egg producers is a great way to find high-quality eggs that are generally fresher and less expensive than the eggs you'll find in a grocery store.

Seafood

Seafood is rich in beneficial proteins and vitamins and minerals, but the most important health benefits related to seafood come from two specific omega-3 fatty acids: eicosapentaenoic acid (EPA) and docosahexaenoic acid (DHA).

Regular consumption of EPA and DHA has been shown to reduce the risk of heart disease, cancer, type 2 diabetes and autoimmune diseases.

When choosing fish, it is best to consume smaller species of fish. Larger fish higher in the food chain tend to accumulate more mercury and other heavy metals and toxins in their meat. Fish and shellfish that are higher in omega-3s include:

- Herring
- Mackerel
- Mussels
- Oysters
- Salmon
- Sardines
- Trout

Wild Rhythms Reared On the Farm

In addition to choosing smaller fish that are rich in omega-3 fatty acids, it is also better to choose fish caught in the wild rather than farmed. As with animals bred for conventional meat, farmed fish receive a diet that is not natural for them. This can include corn and cereals. As a result of their unnatural diet, farmed fish become rich in omega-6 fatty acids and low in omega-3 fatty acids. In fact, according to an analysis published in the Journal of the American Dietetic Association, omega-3 fatty acids could not even be detected in some farm-raised fish found in supermarkets. In addition to the altered levels of fatty acids, farmed fish accumulate higher levels of toxins and contaminants in their meat.

Fruits and Vegetables

You know that fruits and vegetables are good for you. Sure, some fruits contain more natural sugar than others, but when this sugar is combined with the fiber in the fruit, it's not a problem for most people. Problems arise from drinking too much fruit juice, which contains all the sugar without any fiber, so when eating the fruit, be sure to eat it whole and ideally with the skin (which contains fiber).

There is also research showing that organic products not only contain less pesticides and herbicides than conventional products, but are also richer in some vitamins and minerals.

The dirty dozen and fifteen clean

If your budget doesn't allow many organic options, you can prioritize which organic fruits and vegetables to buy using the Environmental Task Force's Dirty Dozen list. The Dozen Dirty list describes which fruits and vegetables have the greatest contamination. These are the products you should prioritize when buying organic products. The dirty dozen (in descending order) are:

- Strawberries
- Spinach
- Nectarines
- Apples

- Grapes
- Peaches
- Cherries
- Pears
- Tomatoes
- Celery
- Potatoes
- Sweet peppers

In addition to the Dirty Dozen list, the Environmental Task Force also provides a list of products that tend to contain the least amount of pesticides and contaminants. These fruits and vegetables are the ones you don't have to prioritize when buying organic products. This list is called Clean Fifteen (starting with the cleanest):

- Avocado
- Sweet corn
- Pineapple
- Cabbages
- Onions
- Frozen sweet peas
- Papayas
- Asparagus
- Mango
- Aubergines
- Honeydew melons
- Kiwi
- Melons
- Cauliflower
- Broccoli

Fats and oils

Fat is nothing to fear. In fact, including healthy fats in the diet can provide you with valuable vitamins and minerals and help you stay full longer. The key is to choose the fats that are good for you. Natural and healthy fats are vital components of a balanced diet.

Margarine contains trans fats in the form of hydrogenated oils. Trans fats were created to give foods a longer shelf life, but have a detrimental effect on cholesterol levels. Unlike saturated fats, which increase large and fluffy LDL particles that do not adhere to the walls of the arteries, trans fats increase the small and dense LDL particles that adhere to the walls of the arteries and can cause blockages that increase the risk of heart disease.

Refined oils such as soybean oil, which is a common ingredient in many prepackaged foods, are rich in omega-6 fatty acids. As you have already learned, eating too many omega-6 fatty acids can contribute to chronic inflammation, which is linked to a variety of diseases and health problems. The best fats to consume include:

- Avocado oil
- Coconut oil
- Grass-fed Ghee
- Hemp oil
- Olive oil
- Sesame oil

- Unsalted grass-fed butter
- Walnut oil

Sugar

Most of the health problems that are often attributed to fat are actually due to sugar. Sugar has no health benefits; however the average American consumes around 66 pounds of sugar per year. Even more worrying than not having any nutritional value is the fact that sugar contributes to chronic inflammation, increases the risk of heart disease, destabilizes blood sugar levels and nourishes cancer cells. Eating too much sugar can also facilitate weight gain.

Manufacturers have attempted to solve the sugar problem by introducing artificial sweeteners on the market, but studies show that people who consume artificial sweeteners have an increased risk of diabetes, metabolic syndrome and heart disease. Artificial sweeteners can also eliminate the balance of bacteria in the intestine, causing both digestive and systemic problems. Artificial sweeteners have even been associated with cancer and chronic migraines. Also, when you give your body the sweet, calorie-free flavor, it can lead to even more intense sugar cravings.

The best options for sweeteners

Regardless of the form it is in, sugar should be limited as much as possible. However, there are some sweeteners that are better for you than others. The best options include:

- Coconut sugar
- Date sugar
- Erythritol (in moderation)
- Molasses
- Fruit of the monk
- Palm sugar
- Pure maple syrup
- Raw honey
- Stevia (in moderation)

Although stevia is a plant and is marketed as natural, many packaged forms are highly elaborate when available. In addition, some Stevia products also contain additional ingredients, such as "natural flavors", which are unfavorable. The term natural flavors is not strictly regulated by the FDA and companies are free to use this description also for chemical additives that mimic natural flavors. If you choose to use stevia, do it in moderation and be sure to choose a pure and organic one.

CHAPTER FIVE-30 Days Intermittent Fasting Plan if you are Busy

Breakfast for your Intermittent Fasting

Breakfast is the most important meal of the day and the same can still be said during the intermittent fasting routine. Breakfast is what gets us going in the morning, so don't deprive yourself! Here in this chapter we will provide you with the meals you need to stay healthy and satisfied throughout the day!

Green Eggs and Bacon

Who needs green eggs and ham when you can eat green eggs and bacon? This recipe is completely loaded with eggs and bacon, as well as avocado, almonds, garlic and an intelligent mixture of spices to keep everything in place.

Preparation time: 5 min.

Passive time: 0 min.

Cooking time: 5 min.

Total: 10 minutes

For 3-4 people

Ingredients:

2 eggs

3 slices of bacon

1 tablespoon of olive oil

1 avocado

1 teaspoon salt

1 teaspoon pepper

1 tbsp pesto

¼ cup of almonds

1 tablespoon of minced basil

1 tablespoon of olive oil

2 tbsp lemon juice

1 tablespoon minced garlic

1 teaspoon of coconut oil

Directions:

1. Take out a medium skillet and add the 2 eggs, the 3 slices of bacon and the spoonful of olive oil.

2. Set the burner over medium heat and mix the ingredients in the oil during cooking for about 2 minutes.

3. Now add the teaspoon of salt, the teaspoon of pepper, the spoon of pesto and the ¼ cup of almonds in the pan.

4. Stir and cook for another 5 minutes.

5. Now place the avocado on a clean cutting board and slice it.

6. Put on a plate, add bacon and eggs and serve!

Morning Casserole

Wake up in the morning with this fantastic saucepan! With eggs, spaghetti, cream and cheddar cheese, this dish has an exceptional flavor!

Preparation time: 5 min.

Passive time: 0 min.

Cooking time: 25 min.

Total: 30 minutes

For 5-6 people

Ingredients:

2 cups of cooked zucchini

12 eggs

1 cup of cream

1 cup of grated cheddar cheese

Directions:

1. Go ahead and set the oven to 375 degrees.

2. While the oven is warming up, remove a bowl and add the 2 cups of cooked pumpkin, 12 eggs, the cup of cream and the cup of grated cheddar cheese.

3. Mix these ingredients well and pour them into a saucepan.

4. Put the dish in the oven and cook the ingredients for about 25 minutes.

5. Serve when ready.

Egg, Vegetable and Beef Omelette

So you say you want to eat well and lose fat? Well, with the right kick of eggs, vegetables and meat, this Omelet has the perfect breakfast!

Preparation time: 2 min.

Passive time: 0 min.

Cooking time: 8 min.

Total: 10 minutes

For 2 people

Ingredients:

2 teaspoons of coconut oil

¼ cup chopped onion

1/2 kg of minced beef

½ cup of grated cooked bacon

½ cup of chopped tomatoes

1 cup of chopped spinach

½ teaspoon salt

1 teaspoon pepper

3 eggs

Directions:

1. First, set the oven to 355 degrees.

2. While the oven is heating up, remove two sheets of aluminum foil.

3. Put a large pan on a stove over high heat and add 2 teaspoons of coconut oil, ¼ cup of chopped onion and ½ kg of minced meat.

4. Mix and cook these ingredients for about 5 minutes.

5. Then add your cup of chopped tomatoes, your cup of chopped spinach and season with ½ teaspoon salt and a teaspoon pepper.

6. Stir and cook for another 3 minutes.

7. After this, take out a medium bowl and add the 3 eggs, stirring.

8. Pour the cooked meat mixture into the medium bowl and mix all the ingredients.

9. Put this combined mixture back into the pan and cook for about 10 minutes on each side.

10. Serve when ready.

Eggs in Limbo

If you need a good and satisfying breakfast in the morning, this dish has it. Loaded with onions, garlic, tomatoes and eggs, you have everything you need to start the day. So don't just fix your plate with akimbo elbows, put a fork and knife in those hands and dive into this underground world of breakfast: eggs in limbo!

Preparation time: 4 min.

Passive time: 0 min.

Cooking time: 8 min.

Total: 12 min.

For 1-2 people

Ingredients:

1 tablespoon of olive oil

½ cup of chopped onion

1 teaspoon minced garlic

1 cup of chopped tomatoes

1 teaspoon pepper

3 tablespoons of minced basil

4 eggs

Directions:

1. Put a medium skillet on a fire over medium heat and add your spoonful of olive oil, followed by ½ cup of chopped onion, your teaspoon of chopped garlic, your cup of chopped tomatoes and your teaspoon of pepper ground.

Almond and Coconut Flour Pancakes

You won't be late for breakfast with this recipe on the menu! You will love the taste of these fantastic pancakes!

Preparation time: 4 min.

Passive time: 0 min.

Cooking time: 4 min.

Total: 8 minutes

For 2-3 people

Ingredients:

½ cup of coconut flour

2 cups of almond flour

1 tbsp sugar

½ teaspoon of baking powder

½ teaspoon of sea salt

1 cup of almond milk

2 tablespoons of butter, melted

1 teaspoon vanilla extract

7 large eggs

Directions:

1. Take out a large bowl and add your half cup of coconut flour, your 2 cups of almond flour, your spoon of sugar, your half teaspoon of yeast and your half teaspoon of sea salt.

2. Now take another bowl and add your 2 cups of almond milk, your 2 tablespoons of melted butter, the teaspoon of vanilla extract and your 7 eggs.

3. Mix this ingredient bowl before adding it to the other ingredient bowl.

4. Mix everything together; This completes your pancake batter.

5. Make a batch of dough for each pancake you make.

6. Place the pancake groups in a large pan and cook 2 minutes on each side over high heat.

7. Serve when ready.

Muesli and Cinnamon

Tired of complex recipes that take too long? Well, if so, for a simple and easy breakfast that requires the minimum, try this tasty batch of muesli and cinnamon! You will be happy to have done it!

Preparation time: 5 minutes and 45 seconds

Passive time: 0 min.

Cooking time: 20 min.

Total: 25 minutes and 45 seconds

For 3-4 people

Ingredients:

2 tablespoons of chia seeds

3 spoons of water

½ teaspoon vanilla extract

½ cup of macadamia nuts

1 tablespoon of whey protein powder

2 tablespoons of flaxseed flour

1 teaspoon cinnamon

½ teaspoon salt

2 tablespoons of melted coconut oil

Directions:

1. Set the oven temperature to 355 degrees.

2. Now take a medium bowl and add your 2 tablespoons of chia seeds, your 3 tablespoons of water and your ½ teaspoon of vanilla extract and mix well.

3. So, take your half cup of macadamia nuts, your tablespoon of whey protein powder, your 2 tablespoons of flaxseed flour, your teaspoon of cinnamon and your half teaspoon of salt and add them to the blender.

4. Blend for about 45 seconds.

5. Put the mixture on a piece of parchment, on a baking sheet and use your (clean) hands to flatten it.

6. Bake and cook for 15 minutes.

7. Remove from the oven and overlap the contents of the other bowl: the chia mixture on top of the ingredients already on the sheet.

8. Return to the oven and cook for another 5 minutes.

9. After 5 minutes, remove the sheet from the oven, cut it into squares and serve.

Bowl of Porridge

As we struggle to get up and move in the morning, many of us are reaching the coffee pot to get a dose of our morning courage. But in addition to coffee, this Bowl of Morning Porridge is also good at giving you the push you need to face your day with confidence!

Preparation time: 5 min.

Passive time: 0 min.

Cooking time: 20 min.

Total: 25 minutes

For 2-3 people

Ingredients:

4 tablespoons of grated coconut

1 tablespoon of oat bran

1 tablespoon of flaxseed flour

½ tablespoon of butter

1 tbsp sugar

1 teaspoon cinnamon

½ cup of cream

1 cup of water

1 teaspoon salt

Directions:

1. Put a small saucepan on a high heat and add your 4 tablespoons of grated coconut, followed by your spoonful of oat bran, your spoonful of flaxseed flour, your half spoonful of butter, the your spoon of sugar, your teaspoon of cinnamon, its half cup of cream, its cup of water and its teaspoon of salt.

2. Stir and stir the entire contents of the pan during cooking for the next 20 minutes.

3. Serve when ready.

A Small Lunch in the Middle

When lunch time comes, don't spoil your fast by looking for fast food! Don't let burgers and fries go to your head (or stomach); Try some of these healthy alternatives! You will love it!

Beefy Green Lettuce Wraps

Meat and all the fixings wrapped in a piece of lettuce! This dish is very good; don't be surprised if you want to dive. Go ahead, prepare this little green for your lunch, friend!

Preparation time: 3 min.

Passive time: 0 min.

Cooking time: 7 min.

Total: 10 minutes

For 3-4 people

Ingredients:

1 tablespoon of olive oil

2 spoons of chopped onion

½ teaspoon minced garlic

1 teaspoon of chilli powder

1 kg of lean ground beef

1 tablespoon of coriander, chopped

1 spoonful of chopped parsley

½ teaspoon of sea salt

1 teaspoon pepper

½ cup of chopped tomatoes

½ cup of chopped cucumbers

1 tbsp lemon juice

½ teaspoon cayenne pepper

½ teaspoon of sea salt

1 cup diced avocado

4 leaves of romaine lettuce

Directions:

1. In a medium skillet, add your spoonful of olive oil, distribute it evenly and put the burner on medium heat.

2. Then add the 2 tablespoons of chopped onion, ½ teaspoon of chopped garlic, the teaspoon of chilli powder and mix and cook for about 2 minutes.

3. Next, add the pound of lean ground beef, stir and cook for another 5 minutes.

4. While cooking, remove a medium bowl and add your tablespoon of chopped parsley, your half teaspoon of sea salt, your teaspoon of pepper, your half cup of chopped tomatoes, your half cup of chopped cucumbers, the your spoonful of lemon juice, your half teaspoon cayenne pepper, your half teaspoon sea salt, your cup of chopped avocado. Mix well.

5. Now go back to your meat mix and place it on the lettuce leaves.

6. Finally, add your mug over the meat, wrap the lettuce leaves and the bags of green lettuce with the meat are done!

Sauteed Mushrooms, Chicken and Vegetables

If you are looking for a good lunch, I have a suggestion: mushrooms, chicken and all your favorite vegetables sauteed to perfection.

Preparation time: 2 min.

Passive time: 0 min.

Cooking time: 8 min.

Total: 10 minutes

For 2 people

Ingredients:

2 teaspoons of coconut oil

1 teaspoon minced ginger

½ teaspoon minced garlic

½ teaspoon hot pepper

1 cup of chopped chicken

½ cup of chopped mushrooms

1 cup of chopped cabbage

½ cup of chopped carrots

½ cup of celery, chopped

½ cup of chopped green pepper

1 tablespoon of coconut oil

1 teaspoon of sea salt

1 teaspoon pepper

1 teaspoon sesame seeds

Directions:

1. In a medium skillet, add the 2 teaspoons of coconut oil and put the burner on a high heat.

2. Now add your teaspoon of minced ginger, your half teaspoon of minced garlic, your half teaspoon of hot pepper and your cup of minced chicken.

3. Stir and cook these ingredients for about 4 minutes, before adding ½ cup of chopped mushrooms and cook for 1 more minute.

4. Then add your cup of grated cabbage, followed by your half cup of celery, your half cup of chopped green pepper, your spoon of coconut oil, your teaspoon of sea salt, your teaspoon of pepper and the your teaspoon of sesame seeds

5. Mix everything and cook in the next 3 minutes.

6. Serve when ready.

Turkey Lettuce Burger

You can take the healthy flavor of the meatloaf and roll it in these delicious turkey lettuce burgers! If you are hungry and need something that fills you well, try this recipe!

Preparation time: 5 min.

Passive time: 0 min.

Cooking time: 5 min.

Total: 10 minutes

For 2 people

Ingredients:

1 kilo of ground turkey

2 egg whites

¼ cup chopped onion

3 spoons of tomato sauce

1 tablespoon minced garlic

¼ teaspoon dried oregano

½ teaspoon salt

2 slices of tomato

4 large lettuce leaves

2 tablespoons of Dijon mustard

Directions:

1. In a medium bowl, add your pound of ground turkey, its 2 egg whites, its ¼ cup of chopped onion, its 3 tablespoons of

chopped garlic, its ¼ teaspoon of dried oregano and the his ½ teaspoon of salt.

2. Now take your (clean) hands and use them to press the ingredients into 2 separate meatballs.

3. Put a medium skillet on a stove over high heat and put your 2 meatballs in the pan.

4. Cook for about 5 minutes on each side.

5. During cooking, place the lettuce leaves on two separate plates.

6. Put the cooked hamburger on one of the sheets and add each with 1 slice of lettuce and 1 tablespoon of Dijon mustard.

7. Now place the remaining sheet on each hamburger.

8. Your turkey lettuce burgers are ready to eat!

Sauté Chicken

You know what they say: a little shaking can really do a lot! And with this delicious dish, this is definitely the case!

Preparation time: 2 min.

Passive time: 0 min.

Cooking time: 8 min.

Total: 10 minutes Servings: 2-3

Ingredients:

• 2 cups of shredded chicken

• 1 tablespoon of soy sauce

• 2 tablespoons of olive oil

• 1 teaspoon of grated ginger

- ½ cup diced green pepper
- 1 cup of cooked rice

Directions:

1. Put a medium pan on a medium-high heat and add 2 tablespoons of olive oil to the pan.

2. Now add your 2 cups of grated chicken followed by your spoonful of soy sauce and your teaspoon of grated ginger.

3. Stir and cook the ingredients for about 5 minutes, before adding ½ cup of diced green pepper and a cup of cooked rice.

4. Mix and cook all the ingredients together for about 3 more minutes.

5. Serve when ready.

Fire Chicken

Chicken breasts, tabasco and sour cream - Set the lunch routine on fire!

Preparation time: 5 min.

Passive time: 0 min.

Cooking time: 45 min.

Total: 50 min Servings: 1-2

Ingredients:

2 chicken breasts

1 cup of sour cream

2 teaspoons of Tabasco sauce

½ teaspoon celery salt

½ teaspoon black pepper

Directions:

1. Adjust the oven to 355 degrees, grease a pan and set it aside.

2. Now take a small bowl and add your cup of sour cream, your 2 teaspoons of Tabasco sauce, your half teaspoon of celery salt and your half teaspoon of black pepper.

3. Mix the ingredients well.

4. Spread the 2 chicken breasts on the baking sheet and pour the sour cream mixture over the chicken breast.

5. Put the pan in the oven and cook for about 45 minutes.

6. Once cooked, remove it immediately from the oven and serve.

Turkey Lettuce Burger

You can take the healthy flavor of the meatloaf and roll it in these delicious turkey lettuce burgers! If you are hungry and need something that fills you well, try this recipe!

Preparation time: 5 min.

Passive time: 0 min.

Cooking time: 5 min.

Total: 10 minutes

For 2 people

Ingredients:

1 kilo of ground turkey

2 egg whites

¼ cup chopped onion

3 spoons of tomato sauce

1 tablespoon minced garlic

¼ teaspoon dried oregano

½ teaspoon salt

2 slices of tomato

4 large lettuce leaves

2 tablespoons of Dijon mustard

Directions:

1. In a medium bowl, add your pound of ground turkey, its 2 egg whites, its ¼ cup of chopped onion, its 3 tablespoons of chopped garlic, its ¼ teaspoon of dried oregano and the his ½ teaspoon of salt.

2. Now take your (clean) hands and use them to press the ingredients into 2 separate meatballs.

3. Put a medium-sized pan over a high heat and place your 2 grills in the pan.

4. Cook for about 5 minutes on each side.

5. During cooking, place the lettuce leaves on two separate plates.

6. Put the cooked hamburger on one of the sheets and add each with 1 slice of lettuce and 1 tablespoon of Dijon mustard.

7. Now place the remaining sheet on each hamburger.

8. Your turkey lettuce burgers are ready to eat!

Dinner After Fasting

If you've ever gone to bed hungry, you know how hard those night hunger pains can be. It is for this reason that the way we end our day during a fast is as important as the way we start. Here, in this chapter, you will find a list of healthy but abundant foods that you can take for dinner after finishing your fast.

Meatloaf Dinner with Cheese

Meatloaf is a classic of the classic and comfortable food, and you will find that this cheese meatloaf dinner is absolutely fantastic!

Preparation time: 5 min.

Passive time: 0 min.

Cooking time: 25 min.

Total: 30 minutes Servings: 1-2

Ingredients:

1 kg of ground beef

¼ cup of chopped onion

1 tablespoon of minced garlic

1 cup of flax flour

2 tablespoons of coconut oil

4 tablespoons of tomato sauce without sugar

1 tablespoon of dried herbs

¼ cup of chopped green pepper

½ cup of grated cheddar cheese

¼ cup of grated Gouda cheese

½ cup of parmesan

Directions:

1. Set the oven to 355 degrees.

2. While the oven is warming up, put your pound of minced meat, ¼ cup of chopped onion, a spoonful of chopped garlic and a cup of flax flour in a large bowl and stir.

3. Now add your 2 tablespoons of coconut oil, your 4 tablespoons of tomato to the unsweetened passata and the spoonful of dried herbs and mix well.

4. Remove a greased kitchen sheet and distribute the ingredients on the bottom.

5. Follow this by placing the ½ cup of grated cheddar cheese and ¼ cup of grated Gouda cheese over the spread of meat.

6. Now sprinkle with ½ cup of parmesan.

7. Bake and cook for about 25 minutes.

8. Cut and serve.

Salted Beef Fillet and Mushrooms

Eating this dish after a fast will not knot the stomach; this salted meat really hits the spot!

Preparation time: 11 min.

Passive time: 0 min.

Cooking time: 9 min.

Total: 20 minutes Servings: 2

Ingredients:

4 cups of cauliflower, chopped

¼ cup of water

½ kg of beef fillet

1 cup of chopped mushrooms

½ teaspoon salt

1 teaspoon of fresh thyme

¼ teaspoon of ground pepper

Directions:

1. In a heat-resistant container, place the 4 cups of chopped cauliflower and ¼ cup of water.

2. Wrap the bowl in a plastic wrap and cook it in the microwave, cooking the ingredients

4 minutes

3. Now place a large pan on a stove over high heat and put the half-kilo fillet of beef in the pan.

4. Then add your cup of chopped mushrooms and cook the meat for about 5 minutes on each side.

5. Season with ½ teaspoon of fresh thyme and ½ teaspoon of salt.

6. Serve meat and mushrooms on a plate and serve with a side of cauliflower.

Pork chop party

Pork chops offer a hearty feast after fasting!

Preparation time: 5 min.

Passive time: 0 min.

Cooking time: 45 min.

Total: 50 min Servings: 2-3

Ingredients:

7 pork chops

½ cup of chopped onion

¼ cup diced tomato

1 teaspoon pepper

1 teaspoon salt

1 tablespoon of olive oil

Directions:

1. Preheat the oven to 390 degrees.

2. Remove a large pan and grease with a spoonful of olive oil.

3. Spread the 7 pork chops on the pan.

4. Now add ½ cup of diced onion and ¼ cup of diced tomato in the cooking pan.

5. Season with a teaspoon of salt and a teaspoon of pepper and put the pan in the oven.

6. Cook for 45 minutes.

7. Once cooked, serve immediately.

Portobello Philly Cheesesteak

Your Philly Cheesesteak stuffed inside a Portobello mushroom!

Preparation time: 5 min.

Passive time: 0 min.

Cooking time: 7 min.

Total: 12 min.

Serves: 4 ingredients:

6 oz. Sliced sirloin steaks

½ teaspoon kosher salt

1 teaspoon black pepper

1 cup of chopped onion

1 cup of chopped green pepper

1 tablespoon of sour cream

2 tablespoons of mayonnaise

2 ounces of cream cheese

3 ounces of grated provolone

4 large Portobello mushrooms

Directions:

1. Set the oven temperature to 400 degrees.

2. While the oven is warming up, remove the 4 large Portobello mushrooms, remove the stems, remove the gills and season the tops with ½ teaspoon kosher salt and a teaspoon of black pepper.

3. Set them aside for a moment, take a large pan and put them on a high heat.

4. Put the 6 ounces of sliced sirloin steaks in the pan and cook for about 2 minutes on each side.

5. Next, add your cup of chopped onion and your cup of chopped green pepper.

6. Mix and cook these ingredients together for another 3 minutes.

7. Next, place the lids of Portobello mushrooms on a greased pan and then evenly pour the cooked ingredients into the 4 lids.

8. Put these stuffed lids in the oven and cook for about 400 degrees.

Chickpeas with Cheese and Chicken Au Gratin

The delicious chickpeas lend themselves to the classic au gratin chicken flavors!

Preparation time: 2 min.

Passive time: 0 min.

Cooking time: 4 min.

Total: 6 min

For 3-4 people

Ingredients:

1 cup of chickpeas

1 cup of grated chicken

1 can of chicken cream

½ cup of water

1 teaspoon of salt

1 teaspoon pepper

1 cup of grated cheddar cheese

Directions:

1. Add your cup of chickpeas and your cup of grated chicken to a medium saucepan, followed by the can of chicken cream, your half cup of water and your teaspoon of salt.

2. Now put the fire on the stove and stir the ingredients as they cook in the next 4 minutes.

3. After 4 minutes, add your cup of grated cheddar cheese, mixing the cheese with the other ingredients for the next 2 minutes.

4. Finally, turn off the heat, season with your teaspoon of pepper and serve.

Soups, Snacks, Side Dishes and Salads

As much as we would like to focus on what we eat for our main course meals, it is sometimes the smaller appetizers and additions that make the difference. Here in this chapter you will find all the best soups, side dishes and salads to consume during the 30-day intermittent rapid challenge.

Homemade Mushroom Cream

How did mom do! Homemade mushroom cream!

Preparation time: 3 min.

Passive time: 0 min.

Cooking time: 20 min.

Total: 23 min

For 1-2 people

Ingredients:

1 tablespoon of coconut oil

1 cup of chopped onion

1 teaspoon minced garlic

½ cup of chopped mushrooms

1 teaspoon of fresh thyme

3 cups of chicken broth

½ cup of coconut milk

½ teaspoon of sea salt

1 teaspoon pepper

Directions:

1. Take out a large saucepan and place it on a high heat.

2. Add your tablespoon of coconut oil, followed by your cup of chopped onion, your teaspoon of chopped garlic, your half cup of chopped mushrooms, your teaspoon of fresh thyme and the 3 cups of chicken broth.

3. Stir and cook all your ingredients together for about 15 minutes, before reducing the heat to medium and adding your half cup of coconut milk, your half teaspoon of sea salt and your teaspoon of pepper.

4. Now stir and cook for another 5 minutes before serving.

Nuts, Crabs and Apples Salad

When people think of salads, they probably consider Caesar and Chicken the best, but this salad of nuts, crabs and apples offers an exceptional flavor: you will be immediately convinced!

Preparation time: 5 min.

Passive time: 0 min.

Cooking time: 0 min.

Total: 5 min Servings: 1-2

Ingredients:

1 cup of crab meat

2 cups of diced unpeeled apples

¼ cup of walnuts

¼ cup of chopped chives

1 tablespoon of chopped dill

2 tablespoons of lemon juice

½ teaspoon salt

1 teaspoon pepper

Directions:

1. Deposit your cup of crab meat, your 2 cups of diced unpeeled apples, your ¼ cup of walnuts, your ¼ cup of chopped chives, your spoonful of chopped dill, your 2 tablespoons of lemon juice, your ½ teaspoon of salt and the teaspoon of pepper.

2. Mix these ingredients lightly and serve when ready.

Rich Fish Soup

You will feel like a million dollars when you eat this soup!

Preparation time: 5 min.

Passive time: 0 min.

Cooking time: 15 min.

Total: 20 minutes

For 1-2 people

Ingredients:

2 teaspoons of olive oil

½ cup of chopped onion

½ teaspoon minced garlic

1 cup diced tomato

¼ cup of chopped carrots

¼ cup diced celery

½ cup of white wine

1 cup of water

¼ teaspoon grated lemon zest

½ pound of fresh cod

¼ teaspoon of sea salt

1 teaspoon pepper

1 tablespoon of chopped parsley

Directions:

1. Add your 2 teaspoons of olive oil in a medium saucepan and put the burner on high heat.

2. Now add ½ cup of chopped onion, ½ teaspoon of chopped garlic, your cup of chopped tomato, your ¼ cup of chopped carrots and your ¼ cup of chopped celery.

3. Stir and cook these ingredients for about 5 minutes before adding ½ cup of white wine and your cup of water to the mixture.

4. Now add ¼ teaspoon of grated lemon zest, followed by your ½ pound fresh cod.

5. Mix everything vigorously for about 10 minutes.

6. Finally, season the mixture with ¼ teaspoon of sea salt, the teaspoon of pepper and the spoonful of chopped parsley.

7. Serve whenever you are ready to do it.

Apple, Cherry and Black Cabbage Salad

Black cabbage salad with the perfect combination of apples and cherries, seasoned to perfection!

Preparation time: 5 min.

Passive time: 0 min.

Cooking time: 0 min.

Total: 5 minutes

For 1-2 people

Ingredients:

1 bunch of cabbage

½ cup of chopped parsley

1 cup of diced apples

½ cup of pitted fresh cherries

¼ cup of shaved red onion

½ teaspoon salt

2 teaspoons of pepper

Directions:

1. Chop the cabbage and put it in a salad bowl.

2. Now add ½ cup of chopped parsley, your cup of diced apples, your ½ cup of fresh chopped cherries, your ¼ cup of shaved red onion, your ½ teaspoon of salt and the 2 teaspoons of bell pepper in the bowl.

3. Mix the ingredients and serve.

Pumpkin Quick and Easy Soup

As the title might suggest, this meal is quick and easy to prepare, but it's also delicious!

Preparation time: 0 min.

Passive time: 0 min.

Cooking time: 0 min.

Total: 0 min Servings: 1-2

Ingredients:

1 tablespoon of olive oil

1 cup of chopped onion

1 cup of chopped pumpkin

2 cups of chicken broth

½ teaspoon nutmeg

¼ teaspoon salt

1 teaspoon pepper

Directions:

1. Put your spoonful of olive oil in a large saucepan, before adding your cup of chopped onion, your cup of chopped pumpkin, your 2 cups of chicken broth, your ½ teaspoon of walnut Muscat, your ¼ teaspoon of salt and your teaspoon of pepper.

2. Mix everything well and cook for 15 minutes on high heat.

3. Serve when ready!

Chinese Chicken Salad

Grilled chicken and Chinese cabbage come together like no other!

Preparation time: 5 min.

Passive time: 0 min.

Cooking time: 0 min.

Total: 5 minutes

Servings: 1-2 Ingredients:

1 cup of chopped chicken breast

4 cups of grated Chinese cabbage

1 cup of peas

1 cup of green bean sprouts

½ cup of grated carrots

½ cup of chopped chives

1 tablespoon of chopped almonds

Directions:

1. Use a fork to destroy your chopped chicken and put it in a medium bowl, followed by your 4 cups of grated Chinese cabbage, your cup of peas, your cup of green bean sprouts, your half cup of grated carrots , your half cup chopped chives and the spoonful of chopped almonds.

2. Mix the salad well and serve it with any type of dressing you want.

Thick and chunky Salsa

Bring out the chips, because this sauce is ready to dip!

Preparation time: 0 min.

Passive time: 0 min.

Cooking time: 0 min.

Total: 0 min Servings: 2-3

Ingredients:

½ cup of chopped onion

1 tablespoon of minced garlic

¼ cup of chopped jalapeño

½ cup of chopped tomatoes

1 teaspoon of coriander

1 tablespoon of lime juice

¼ teaspoon kosher salt

Directions:

1. Take out a blender and add ½ cup chopped onion, 1 tablespoon chopped garlic, ¼ cup chopped jalapeño, ½ cup chopped tomatoes, 1 teaspoon coriander, 1 tablespoon lime juice and ¼ teaspoon kosher salt.

2. Now push the ingredients into the blender 4 or 5 times, so that it mixes but is still nice and thick.

3. After doing so, pour the sauce into a bowl and serve.

Special Desserts and Drinks for Your Fast

Even during the 30 day intermittent quick plan, there will be times when you want something a little more special. There will be times when you want to enjoy a tasty dessert or a drink.

Here in this chapter, we offer several healthy and tasty dessert and drink recipes for your fast.

Cookies with Nuts

Crunchy biscuits with a pinch of hazelnut!

Preparation time: 5 min.

Passive time: 1 min.

Cooking time: 15 min.

Total: 21 min

For 3-4 people

Ingredients:

1 cup of oatmeal

½ cup of chopped hazelnuts

½ cup of white rice flour

½ teaspoon of baking powder

2 sticks of unsalted butter

2 spoons of sugar

3 tablespoons of raspberry jam

1 egg

Directions:

1. Set the oven temperature to 350 degrees and place the parchment on a baking sheet.

2. While the oven is warming up, remove a medium bowl and add your cup of oatmeal, your half cup of chopped hazelnuts, and your half cup of white rice flour and your half teaspoon of yeast, mixing the ingredients well.

3. Now take a separate bowl and add your 2 unsalted butter sticks and 2 spoons of sugar, mixing these ingredients with an electric mixer.

4. Then add the egg and beat with your electric mixer.

5. Now take your bowl of the oatmeal mix and pour it into the bowl of the egg mix.

6. Mix these ingredients with your electric mixer until a uniform mass is formed.

7. Now take a scoop of ice cream and use it to extract bunches of pasta and put them on the baking tray.

8. Put the pan in the oven and cook for about 15 minutes.

9. Once cooked, allow to cool for about 1 minute before serving.

Chocolate Cookies

You will enjoy every chip!

Preparation time: 5 min.

Passive time: 30 seconds

Cooking time: 55 min.

Total: 1 hour and 30 seconds

For 3-4 people

Ingredients:

4 eggs

3 tablespoons of brown sugar

1 tablespoon of normal sugar

8 tablespoons of butter

2 teaspoons of vanilla extract

3 tablespoons of wheat flour for all uses

½ cup of gluten flour

2 tablespoons of raw wheat bran

1 teaspoon of baking powder

½ cup of a whole meal almond flour

½ cup of chocolate chips

¼ cup of chopped walnuts

Directions:

1. Go ahead and set the oven to 350 degrees.

2. While the oven is heating up, take out a medium bowl and add the 4 eggs, 3 tablespoons of brown sugar and the spoonful of normal sugar, take a whisk and mix well.

3. Now add your 8 tablespoons of butter, your 2 teaspoons of vanilla extract, your 3 tablespoons of wheat flour for all uses, your half cup of gluten flour, your 2 tablespoons of wheat bran raw, your teaspoon of baking powder, your half cup of wholemeal almond flour and start beating the mixture once again.

4. Finally, mix the chocolate chips and walnuts in the mixture; put them in the refrigerator and leave to cool for about 45 minutes.

5. After 45 minutes, remove from the refrigerator and use your (clean) hands to form the cookie dough into balls.

6. Distribute these dumplings evenly on a greased pan.

7. Bake for about 10 minutes.

8. Leave to cool for about 30 seconds and serve!

Cream Cheese Cake

Get ready to cook, because this cream cheese fits perfectly with this cream cheese!

Preparation time: 5 min.

Passive time: 0 min.

Cooking time: 30 min.

Total: 35 minutes

For 6-8 people

Ingredients:

20 ounces of cream cheese

4 eggs

2 teaspoons of lemon juice

2 teaspoons of vanilla extract

1 tablespoon of whole wheat flour

½ cup of sour cream

Directions:

1. Set the oven to 325 degrees.

2. While the oven heats up, remove a medium bowl and add 20 ounces of cream cheese and your 4 eggs and use a whisk to whisk the ingredients into a smooth dough.

3. Pour this dough into a spring-shaped pan and place it in your oven.

4. Cook for about 30 minutes.

5. Serve when ready.

Coconut Macaroons

Another big batch of biscuits that tastes great but won't bother you quickly!

Preparation time: 5 min.

Passive time: 30 seconds

Cooking time: 10 min.

Total: 15 minutes and 30 seconds

For 4-5 people

Ingredients:

4 eggs

2 tablespoons of brown sugar

4 tablespoons of butter

2 teaspoons of vanilla extract

2 teaspoons of grated lemon zest

1 tablespoon of wheat gluten flour

1 tablespoon of whole wheat flour

1 teaspoon of baking powder

2 cups of dried coconut

½ cup of whole meal almond flour

Directions:

1. Set the oven temperature to 350 degrees.

2. While the oven is heating, remove a medium bowl and set aside the 4 eggs, 2 tablespoons of brown sugar and 4 tablespoons of butter.

3. Use an electric mixer to blend these ingredients into uniform dough.

4. Then add the 2 teaspoons of vanilla extract, the 2 teaspoons of grated lemon zest, the spoon of wheat gluten flour, the spoon of whole wheat flour and the teaspoon of baking powder, also mixing these ingredients in the 'dough.

5. Now take your (clean) hands and use them to fold the 2 cups of dry coconut and ½ cup of whole meal almond flour.

6. Once this is done, take a scoop of ice cream and use it to collect the dumplings.

7. Spread these dumplings on the surface of a greased pan and put them in the oven.

8. Cook for about 10 minutes, remove, and leave to cool for 30 seconds and serve.

References

Can I Eat Oatmeal on a Candida Diet? | Livestrong.com. https://www.livestrong.com/article/327538-can-i-eat-oatmeal-on-a-candida-diet/

Gym Exercising and Diet Tips - Answers. https://www.answers.com/Q/gym_exercising_and_diet_tips

Herbalife - Ghana - Eating For Energy. https://healthyliving.herbalifeghana.com/articles/eating-well/eating-for-energy

Here's the most important thing you can do to beat COVID-19. https://www.dallasnews.com/opinion/editorials/2020/03/17/heres-the-most-important-thing-you-can-do-to-beat-covid-19/

How God Can Help Those Going Through Emotional Affairs .... https://www.beliefnet.com/love-family/relationships/affairs-and-divorce/how-god-can-help-those-going-through-emotional-affairs.aspx

Measurement Guide - Promlily Online. https://www.promlily.com/measurement-guide.html

No-Knead Multigrain Bread | From Cardamom & Coconut.
https://cardamomandcoconut.com/no-knead-multigrain-bread/

Oven Baked Ribs | Small Town Woman.
https://www.smalltownwoman.com/dry-rub-baked-ribs/

Relaxation: What Happens to Your Body When You actually....
https://www.besthealthmag.ca/best-you/wellness/relaxation/

Printed in Great Britain
by Amazon